MEDITERRANEAN STYLE RECIPES

SUITABLE FOR PESCATARIAN DIET

by Josephine Fandan

TABLE OF **CONTENTS**

TABLE OF **CONTENTS**

TABLE OF **CONTENTS**

Introduction

In this book, you will find Mediterranean-style recipes: couscous, pasta, fish.

Following the Mediterranean diet could bring vast advantages to you. It is excellent for improving energy, protecting your heart, losing weight. Studies have shown that it significantly expands life prospects thanks to its nutrient-rich nature. It can help you to develop your overall well-being.

What makes the eating habits of the Mediterranean people such a famous diet plan is that it's not just the food; it's an entire lifestyle! It is enjoying choosing fresh ingredients only, enjoying cooking, and most importantly enjoy eating tasty and flavorsome meals.

In the book, you will find different recipes to make your tastebuds tingle and make your friends and family go excited! The Mediterranean Diet is the ideal go for a healthy option that is easy to follow.

This diet will give you innumerable options for delicious meals every single day, without the need to count one single calorie.

All recipes are vegetarian and proper for the pescatarian diet as well.

The images do not represent exactly the meal from the recipe.

The measurement used in the recipes:
1 cup is 4.5 oz or 128 grams approximately dry goods
1 cup is 12 oz or 340 grams approximately of liquid

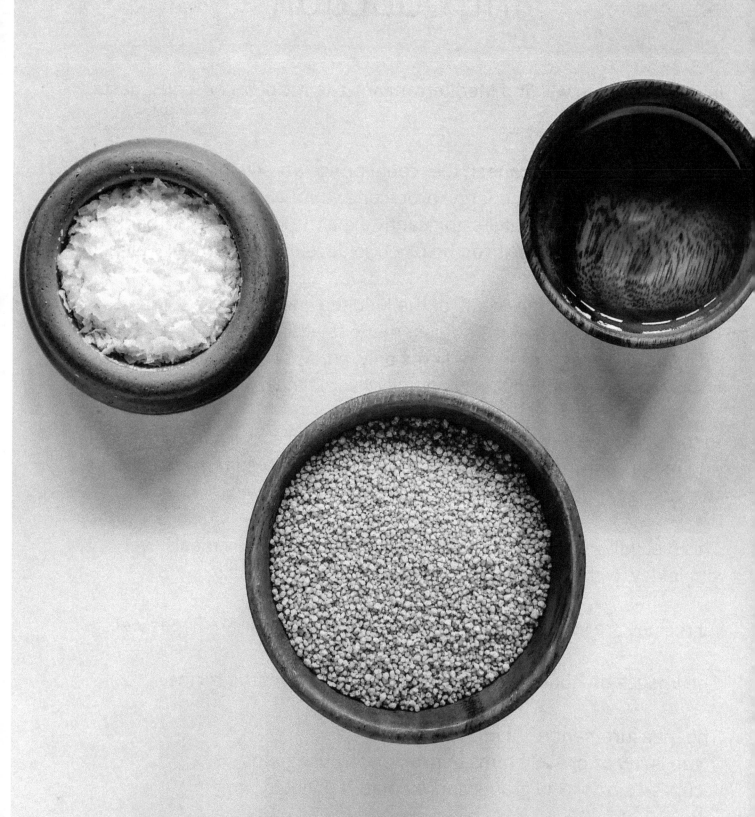

COUSCOUSE BASE RECIPE

INGREDIENTS

1 cup couscous,

2 cups water,

salt,

olive oil

SERVINGS 4
READY IN 20 MIN

INSTRUCTIONS

Fry couscous in a pan with olive oil, stir all the time with a wooden spoon until it changes the color; put the couscous in a bowl through over salted boiling water and cover. You can boil in the water Rosemary or thyme or some aromatic leaves if you want to.

Wait for around 15 min so the couscous will absorb all water and double the volume.

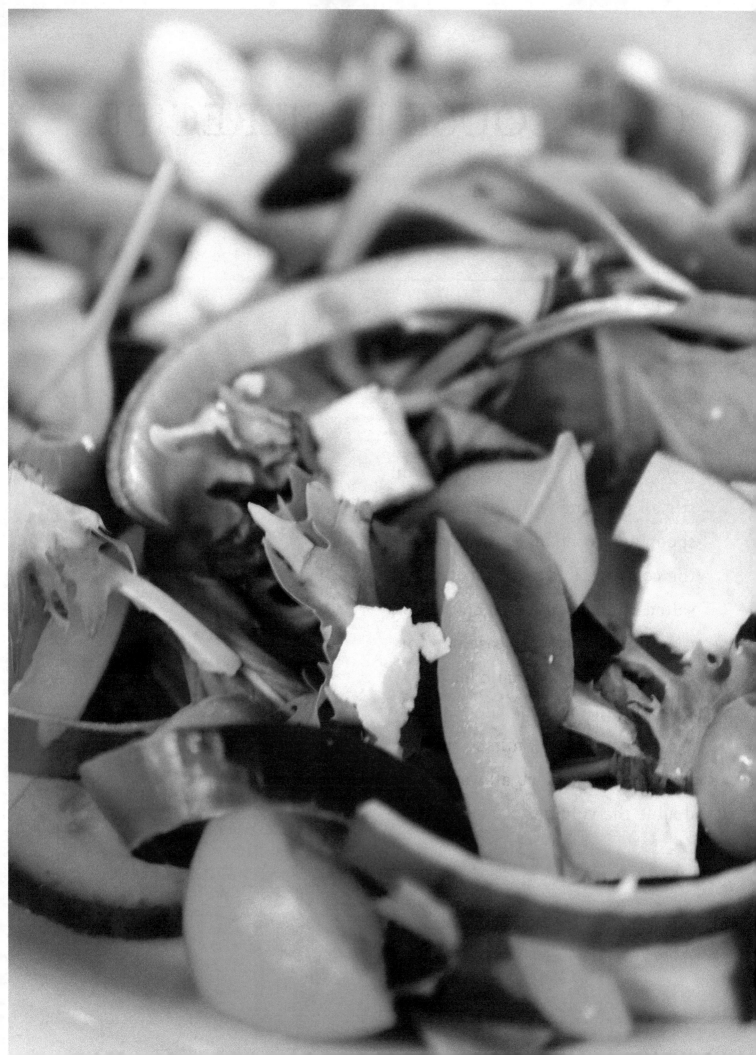

FRESH SALAD

INGREDIENTS

SERVINGS 4
READY IN 10 MIN

juice of 2 lemons
1/4 cup extra-virgin olive oil
salt and freshly ground black pepper to
taste
1 cup cucumbers, diced
4 tomatoes
1/4 cup chopped fresh mint
1/4 cup chopped fresh parsley
4 green onions, sliced thinly

INSTRUCTIONS

Mix all ingredients together in a
serving bowl.

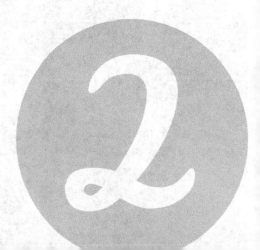

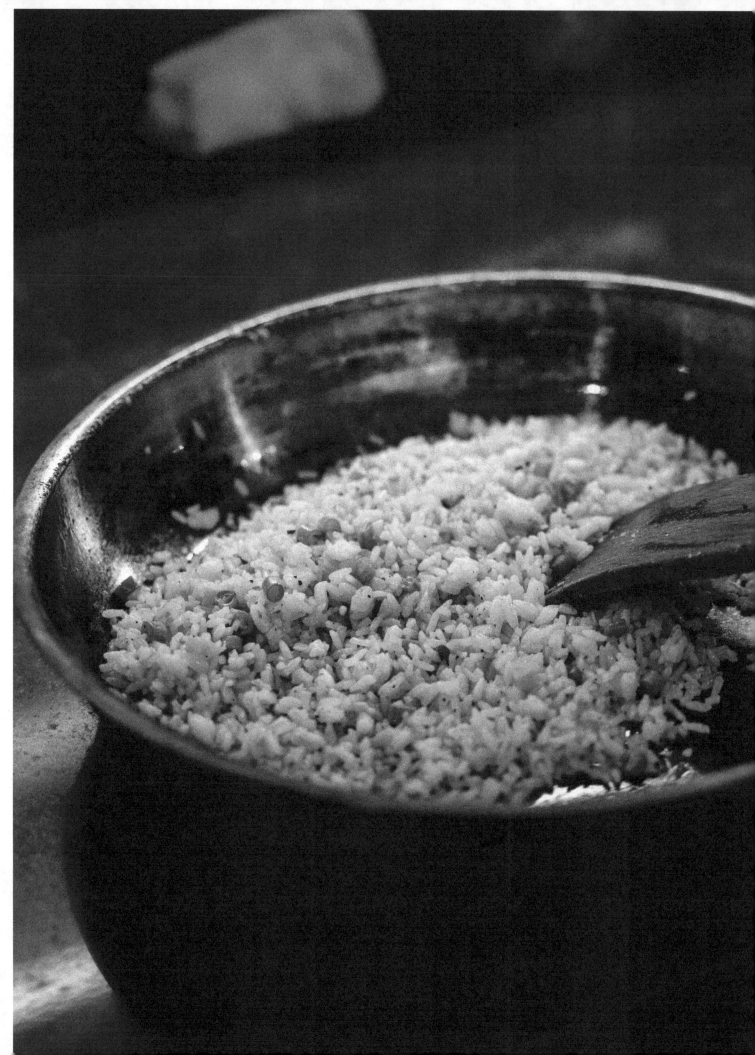

COUSCOUS WITH TOMATOES

INGREDIENTS

SERVINGS 4
READY IN 25 MIN

300 g couscous
4 tomatoes
1 bunch of Persil,
1 tsp cumin seeds,
some leaf of mint,
olive oil,
salt

INSTRUCTIONS

Prepare couscous as described in the base
recipe.
Put the cuscus on a serving plate.
Wash, dry, and cut the tomatoes in slices
and put on couscous, chop Persil and mint,
and mix in the cuscus.

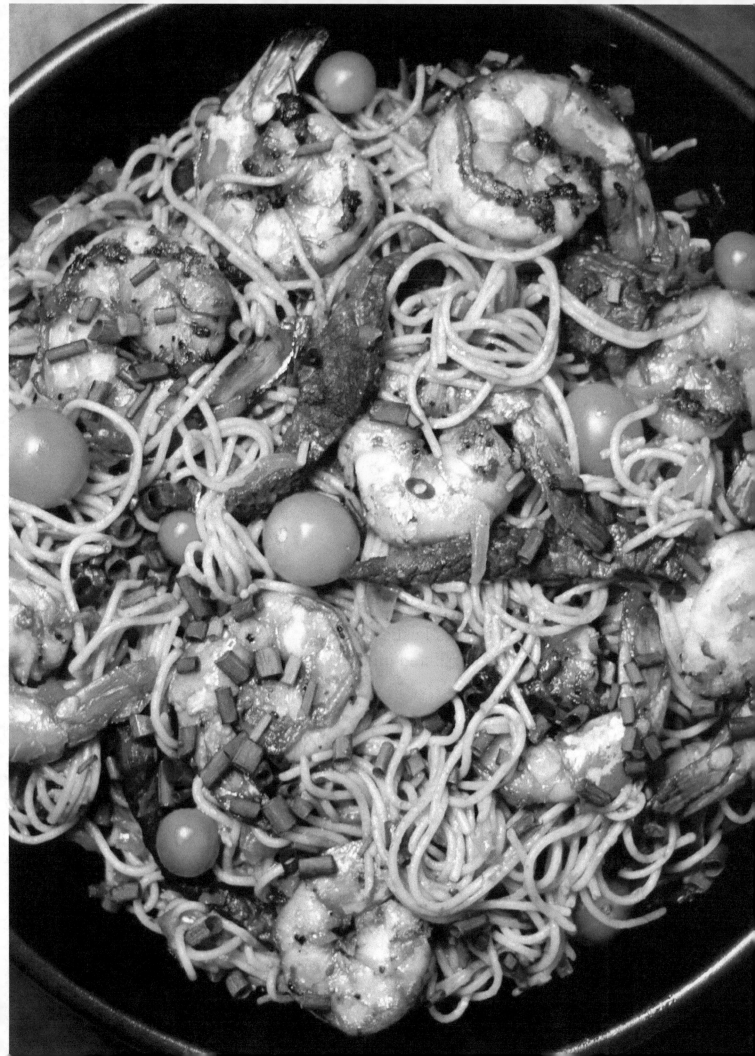

COUSCOUS WITH ROSEMARY

INGREDIENTS

300 g couscous
600 g water
2 tbsp of soy sauce
rosemary
olive oil
salt

SERVINGS 4
READY IN 25 MIN

INSTRUCTIONS

Toasty cuscus with oil and rosemary, as described in the base recipe.
Boil water with soy sauce. Put the cuscus in the bowl through boiling water and cover. Leave for 15 min. Serve on a plate, ideally with vegetables.

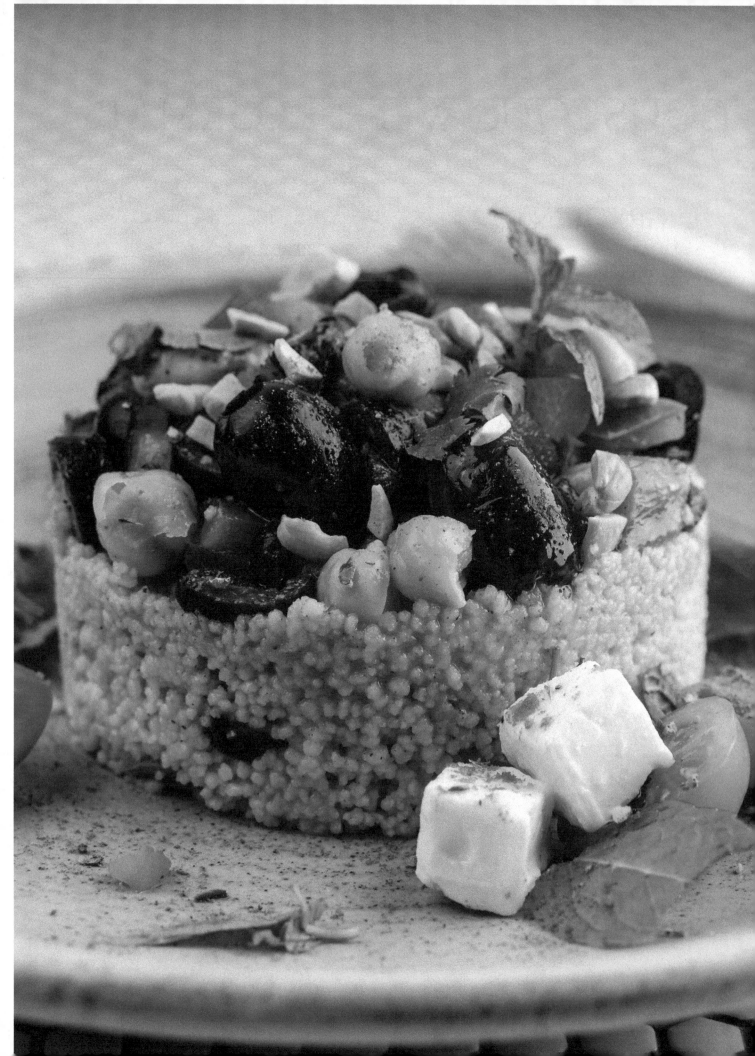

COUSCOUS WITH VEGETABLES

INGREDIENTS

SERVINGS 4

READY IN 20 MIN

300 g couscous
2 onions,
3 carrots,
2 courgettes
2 garlic cloves,
rosemary,
olive oil,
salt

INSTRUCTIONS

Wash and cut long way carrots and courgettes. Cut the onion and fry them in a pan with oil until soft, add carrots, and after 5 min, add courgettes.
In the end, add finely cut garlic and rosemary, and salt, cover the pan, and let on medium heat for 15 min.
Make ready cuscus as in the base recipe. Stir couscous with vegetables and serve.

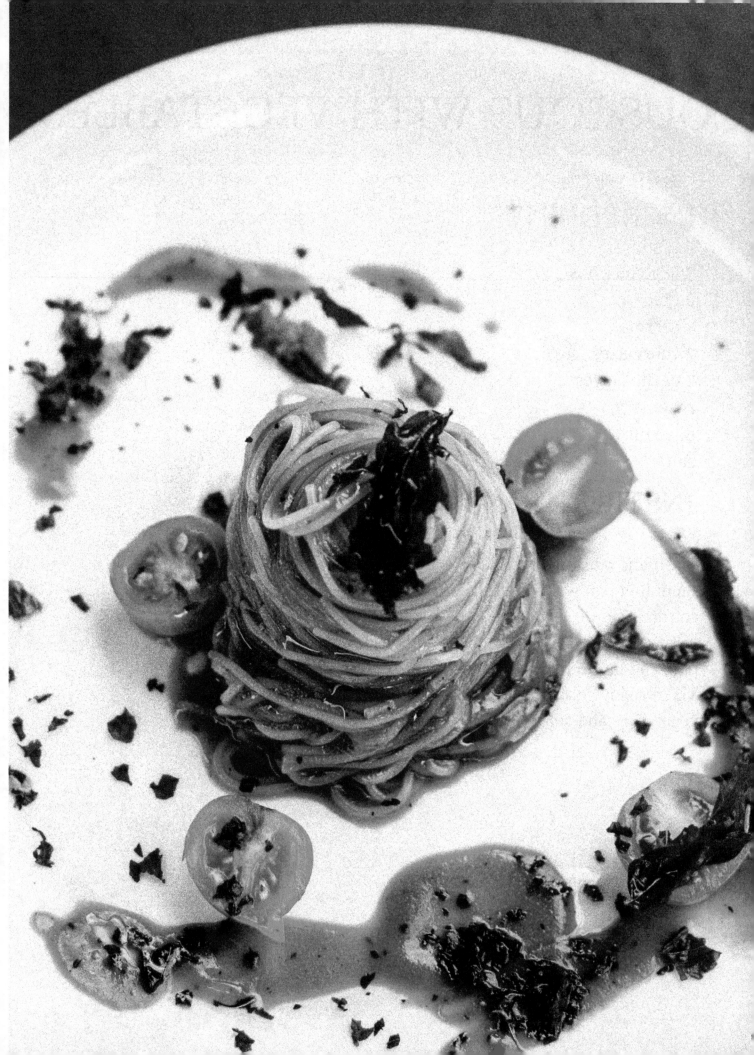

PASTA CARBONARA WITH VEGETABLES

INGREDIENTS

SERVINGS 4
READY IN 25 MIN

400 g pasta
6 small courgettes,
1 onion,
half red pepper
1 leaf cabbage,
2 eggs,
nutmeg,
Parmigiano Reggiano cheese,
olive oil
salt

INSTRUCTIONS

Wash and cut on small pieces the vegetable, fry them in the oil, start with onion, pepper, cabbage leaf, and courgette; after adding salt, cover and let them fry on medium heat for 15 min.

In the meantime, boil pasta in a big pot with salted water. In one bowl, whisk eggs with nutmeg.

After the pasta is boiled, drain and mix the pasta in the pan with vegetables, add a few spoons of olive oil and eggs and let them mix well for 2 minutes on medium heat. Serve with parmigiano reggiano grated cheese on top.

6

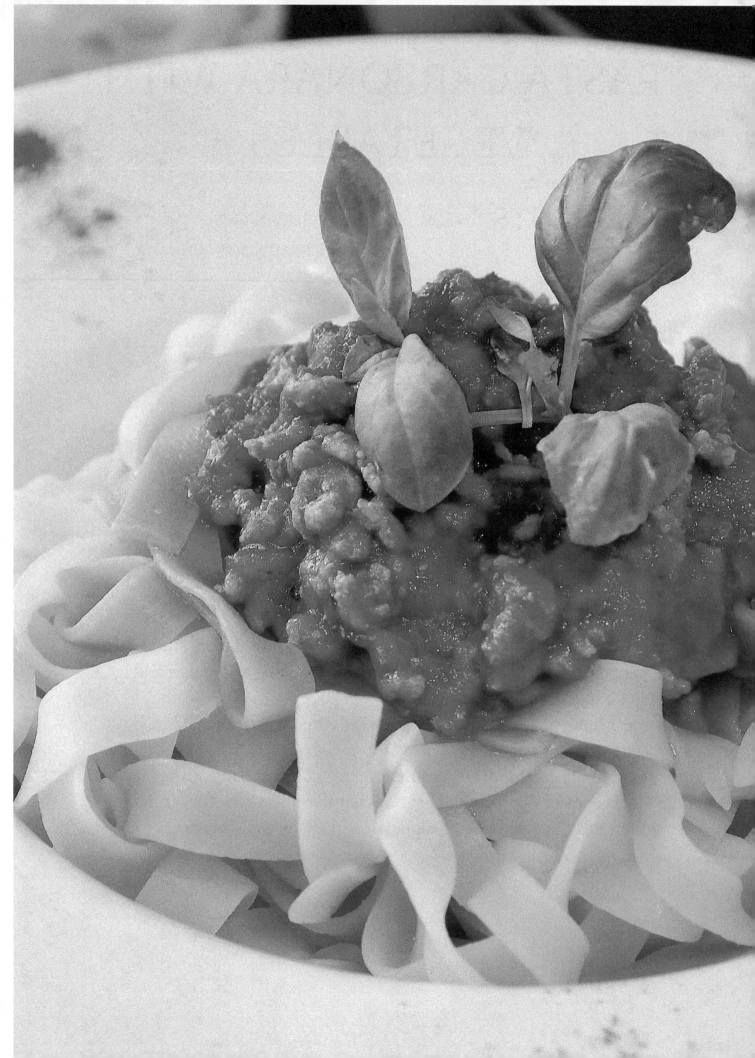

BASIL PASTA

INGREDIENTS

SERVINGS 4

READY IN 20 MIN + macerate
a few hours

400 g of pasta,
1 bunch of fresh basil,
2 cloves of garlic,
150 g green olives,
100 g of grated Parmesan cheese,
olive oil,
salt

INSTRUCTIONS

Finely chop garlic, basil and olives. Then put everything to
macerate in oil for about a couple of hours. Boil the pasta in
plenty of salted water, drain and pour into the bowl in which you
have macerated the sauce; add the grated Parmesan cheese, a
little of the oil, mix well and serve.

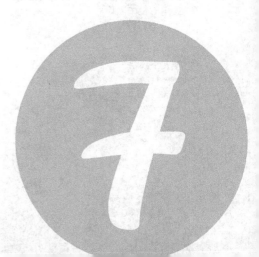

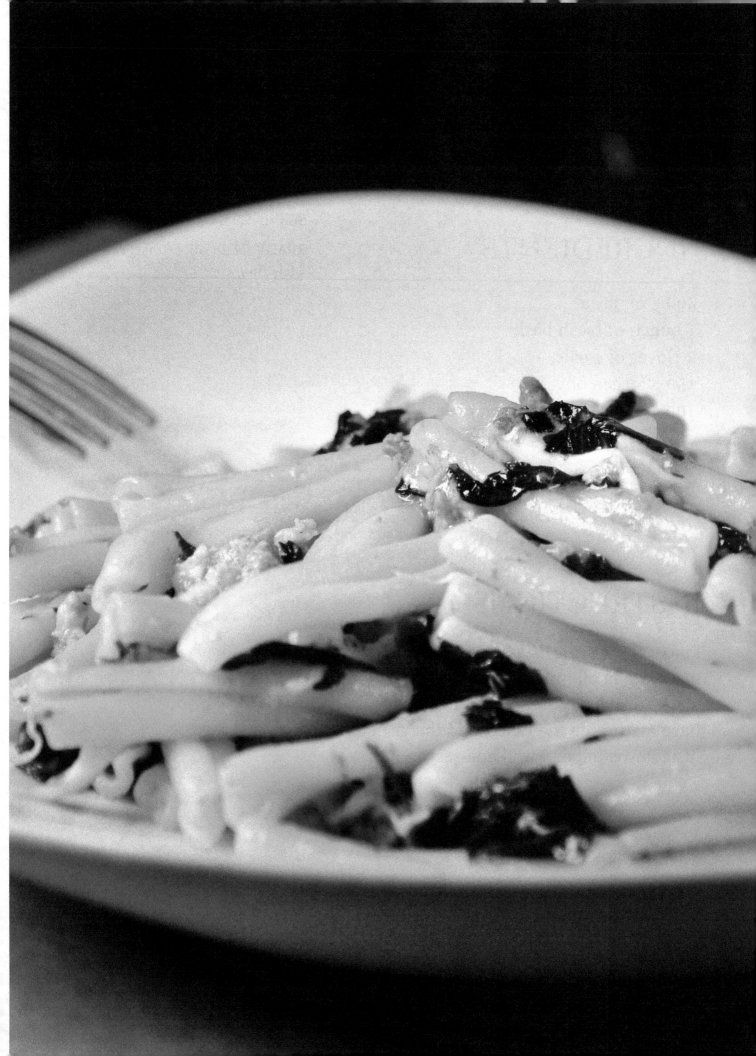

PASTA WITH RICOTTA AND BROCCOLETTI

INGREDIENTS

SERVINGS 4
READY IN 20 MIN

400 g of pasta,
150 g of fresh ricotta,
150 g of broccoli,
1/2 onion,
olive oil,
salt

INSTRUCTIONS

Clean and wash the broccoli and cook them together with the pasta. Meanwhile, sauté the finely sliced onion separately in a bit of oil over low heat. After about ten minutes of cooking, add the ricotta and let it melt, stirring gently. Drain the boiled pasta, and add it to the sauce.

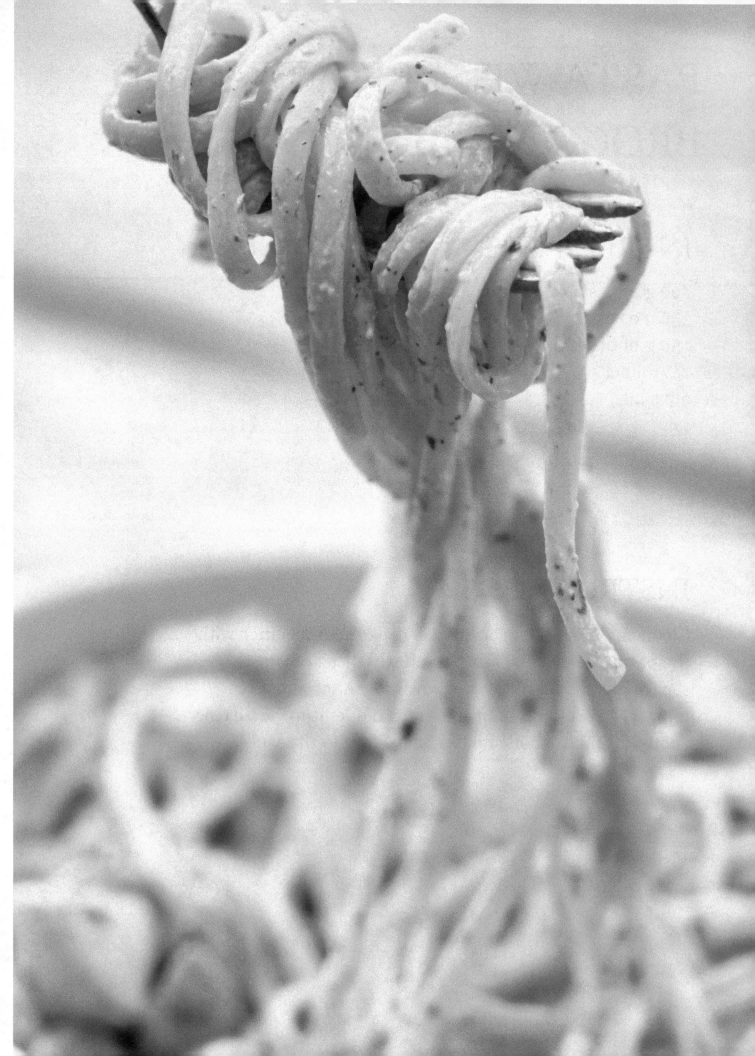

PASTA AND CHICKPEAS

INGREDIENTS

SERVINGS 4

READY IN 1,20 h + soak for 24 hours

300 g of pasta,
150 g of chickpeas,
1 sprig of rosemary,
2 cloves of garlic,
4 tomatoes,
bunch of parsley,
red chili powder,
2 tbsp of soya,
1 tbsp of cumin or fennel seeds,
oil olive, salt

INSTRUCTIONS

Wash the chickpeas, leave them to soak for 24 hours. Drain them, put them in a pot with enough water, and cover; add the rosemary, cumin, or fennel seeds and the peeled tomatoes, let them boil over low heat. Halfway through cooking, remove the rosemary. When cooked, let the chickpeas rest over the heat.
Boil the pasta in salted water and drain. Add it to the legumes and leave it on the fire for a few moments. Divide the food among the plates, add the oil and a pinch of red pepper, soya sauce, and finely chopped garlic cloves and parsley.

9

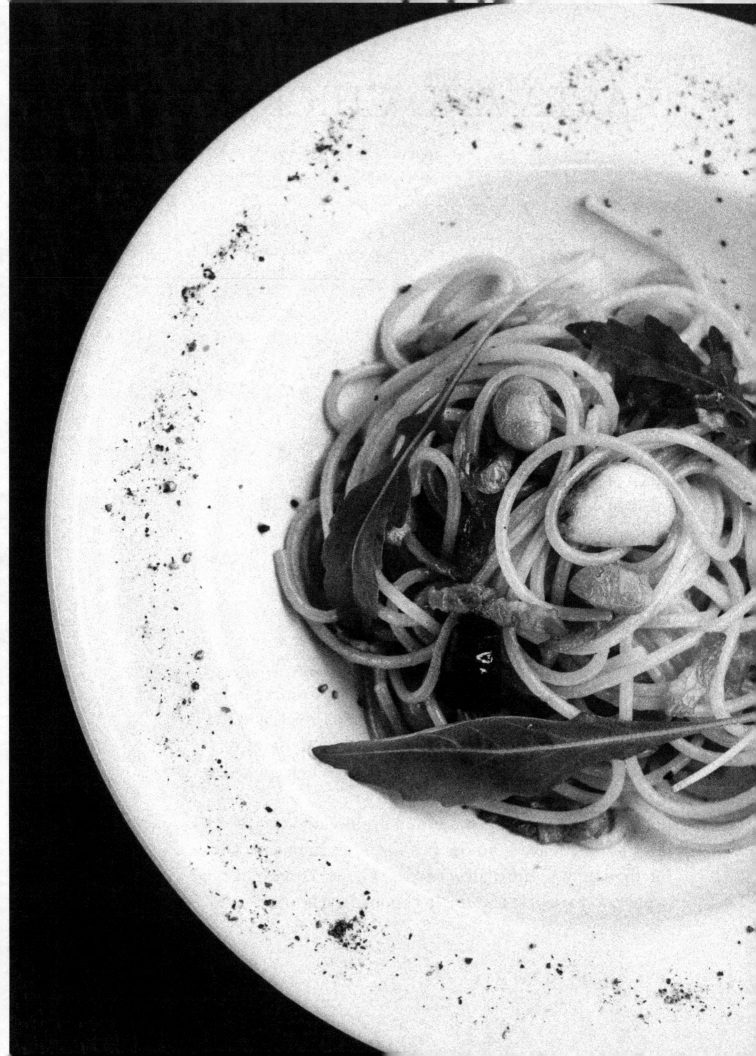

PASTA WITH TURNIP TOP

INGREDIENTS

SERVINGS 4
READY IN 20 MIN

400 g of pasta,
400 g of turnip greens,
100 g of grated Parmesan cheese,
4 cloves of garlic,
1 boned anchovy,
olive oil, salt

INSTRUCTIONS

Clean and cut the pieces of turnip greens and then boil
them in plenty of salted water. Drain, keep the water,
and boil the pasta in that same water. When pasta is
boiled, drain it and mix it with the turnip greens in a
large pan and sauté with oil and finely chopped garlic
for a few minutes. Add Parmigiano Reggiano at the end.

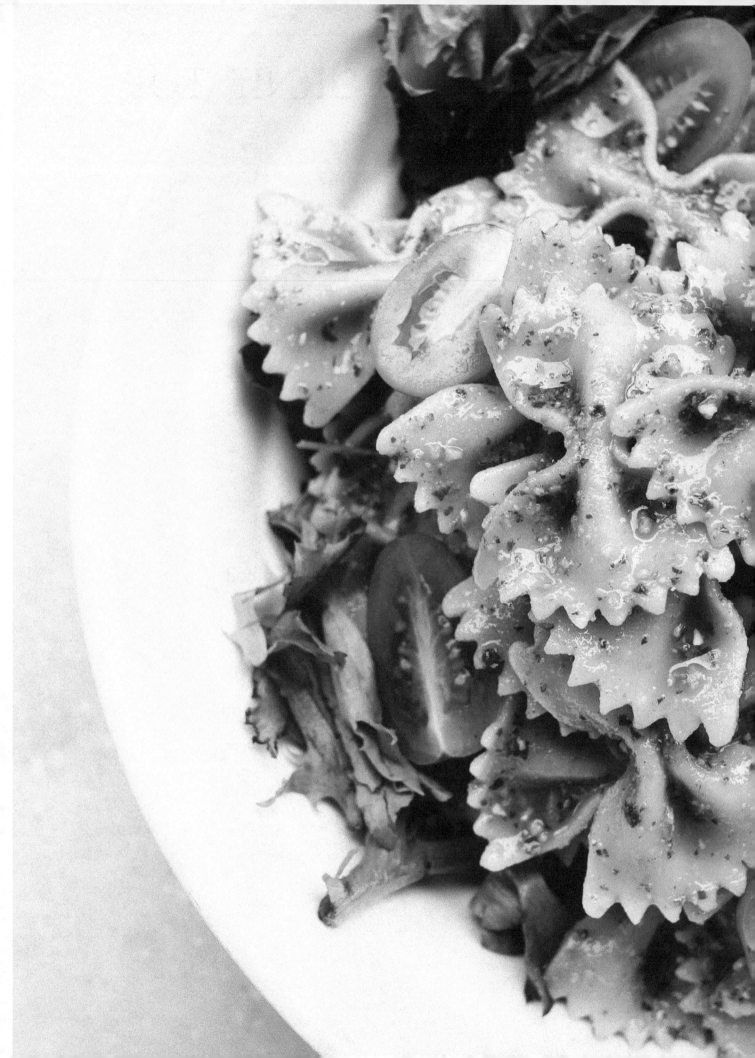

CAULIFLOWER PASTA

SERVINGS 4
READY IN 20 MIN

INGREDIENTS

400 g of pasta,
1 onion,
1 small cauliflower,
80 g of raisins,
80 g of pine nuts,
red chili powder,
grated parmesan,
olive oil,
salt

INSTRUCTIONS

Clean the cauliflower, boil them in salted water, dry it and keep the water. Cut the cauliflower into small pieces. Chop the onion and toss in a pan with a bit of oil, then add the cauliflower, the raisins previously soaked in warm water, the pine nuts, a pinch of chili, and salt, and fry for a few minutes. While the sauce is fry over moderate heat, boil the pasta in the water of the cauliflower. Drain boiled pasta and pour it into the pan with the sauce, mixing it all and adding Parmesan cheese.

11

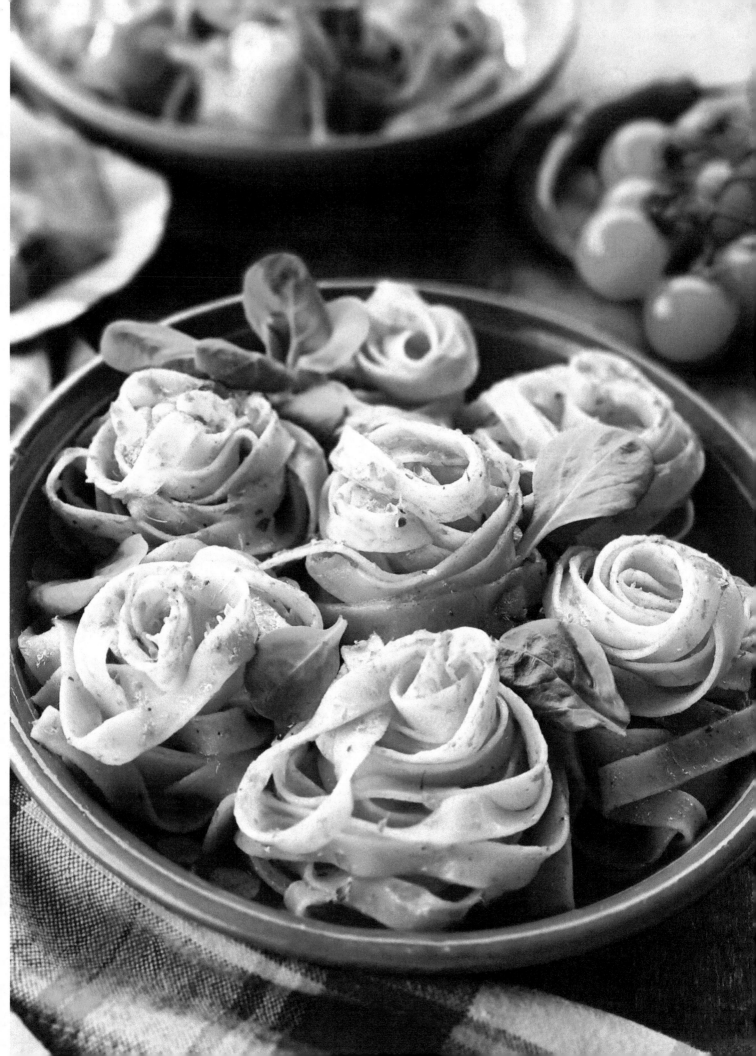

PASTA WITH WALNUTS

INGREDIENTS

SERVINGS 4
READY IN 20 MIN

350 g of noodles
1/2 cup of cooking cream
a handful of walnuts
100 g of fresh cheese
salt

INSTRUCTIONS

Boil the noodles in a pot with plenty of salted
water.
In a saucepan, melt the chopped cheese
together with the cream over low heat. Mix
until well blended, and add the cut walnuts
kernels.
Mix pasta and sauce when everything is still
hot and serve.

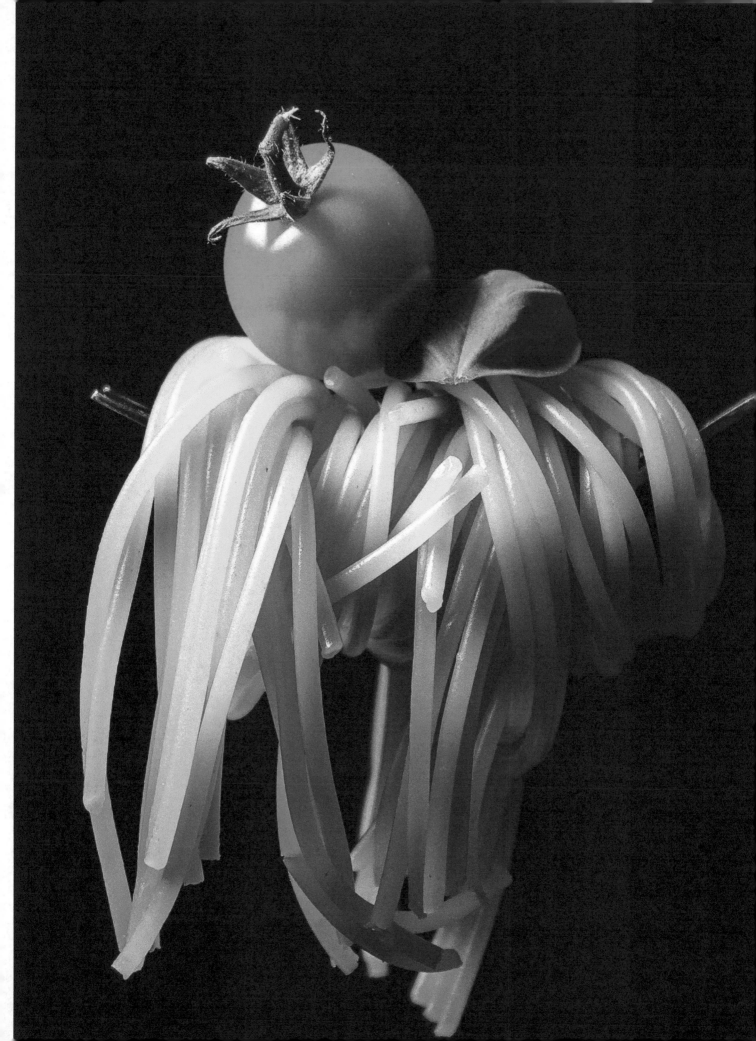

WALNUTS PASTA

INGREDIENTS

320 g of spaghetti,
30 g of walnut kernels
30 g of basil
2 tbsp of grated Parmesan cheese
150 g of ripe cherry tomatoes,
olive oil,
salt and pepper

INSTRUCTIONS

Coarsely chop the walnut kernels and toast everything in a non-stick pan.
Combine the walnuts, the chopped basil, the cheese, a little salt, ground pepper, and 4 tbsp of oil in the blender until creamy pesto.
Cut the cherry tomatoes into wedges.
Mix the spaghetti boiled al dente with the pesto, add the cherry tomatoes, mix and serve.

13

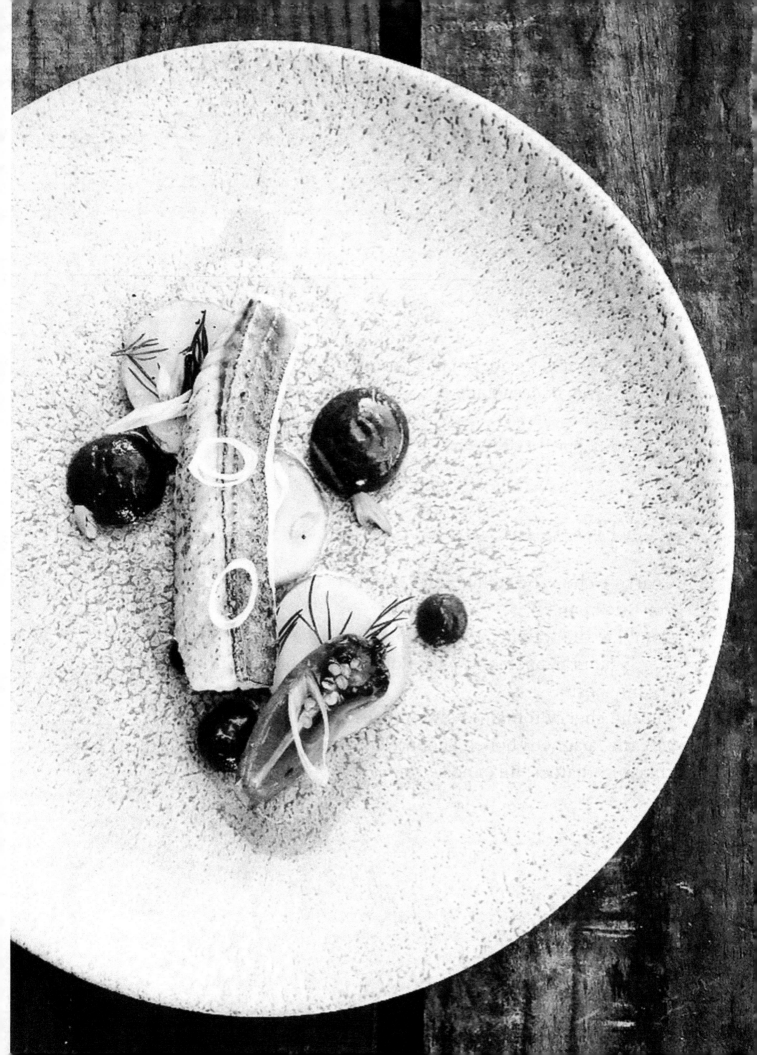

RICE SALAD

INGREDIENTS

320 gr of rice,
100 gr of pickles,
200 gr of tuna in oil,
100 gr of cheese of your choice,
2 eggs,
2 tbsp of olives,
mayonnaise,
extra virgin olive oil

SERVINGS 4

READY IN 20 MIN + 1hour to coll down

INSTRUCTIONS

Cut the pickles into tiny pieces. Cut a cheese of your choice into small cubes. Boil the eggs for 10 minutes. Boil the rice in hot, salted water for the time indicated on the package. Once cooked, drain it, pass it under a large jet of cold water to cool it, transfer it to a big salad bowl, and immediately add a little oil to prevent it from sticking.
Add the drained and chopped tuna, the pickles, the pitted olives, mix and place in a container. Let it cool for an hour. Add the chopped cheese, boiled eggs, and mayonnaise with olive oil when the rice is cold, and mix everything well.

14

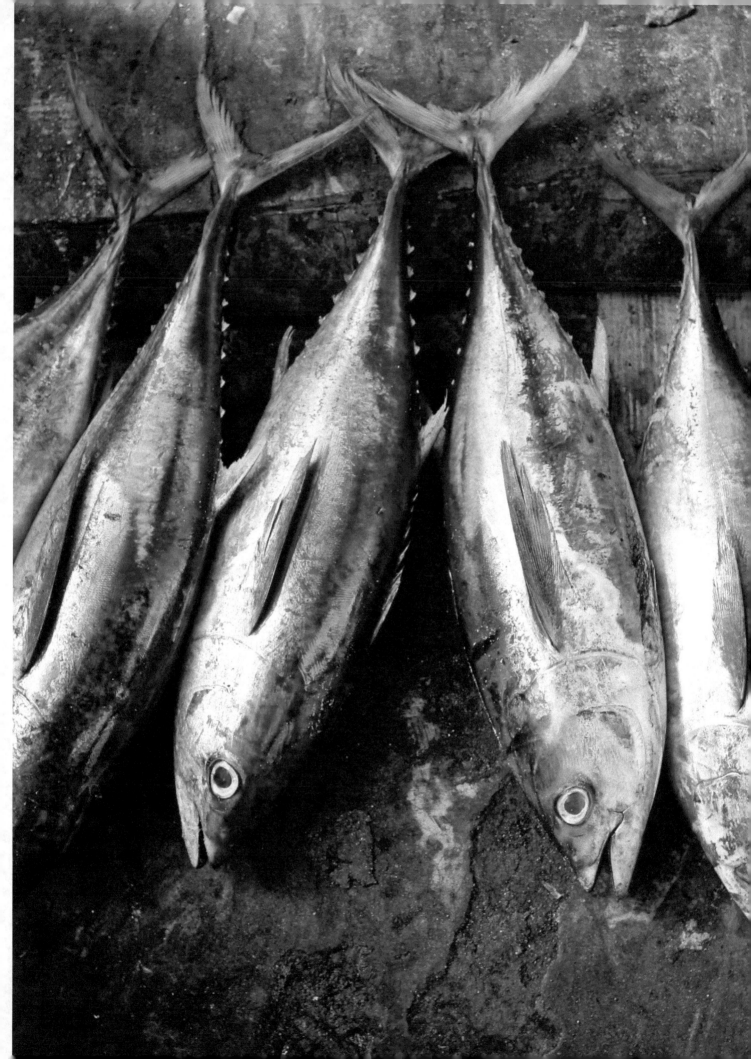

PIKE WITH WINE

INGREDIENTS

SERVINGS 4
READY IN 40 MIN

1 kg - 2 pike
50 g butter
2 leeks
1 carrot
1 stalk of celery
thyme
Laurel
parsley
Flour
1/2 bottle of rose wine
1/2 cup of cream
salt and pepper

INSTRUCTIONS

Wash and clean the fish, cut them into pieces, flour them, and brown them in the pan with butter and a few tbsp of oil. When done, take it out of the pot and keep it aside.

Meanwhile, clean the vegetables and aromatic herbs and chop everything. Fry the chopped vegetable for a few minutes in a pan with oil, add wine, pepper, salt, and cream, and cover for 15 min. Put the sauce over the pieces of the fish and serve hot.

15

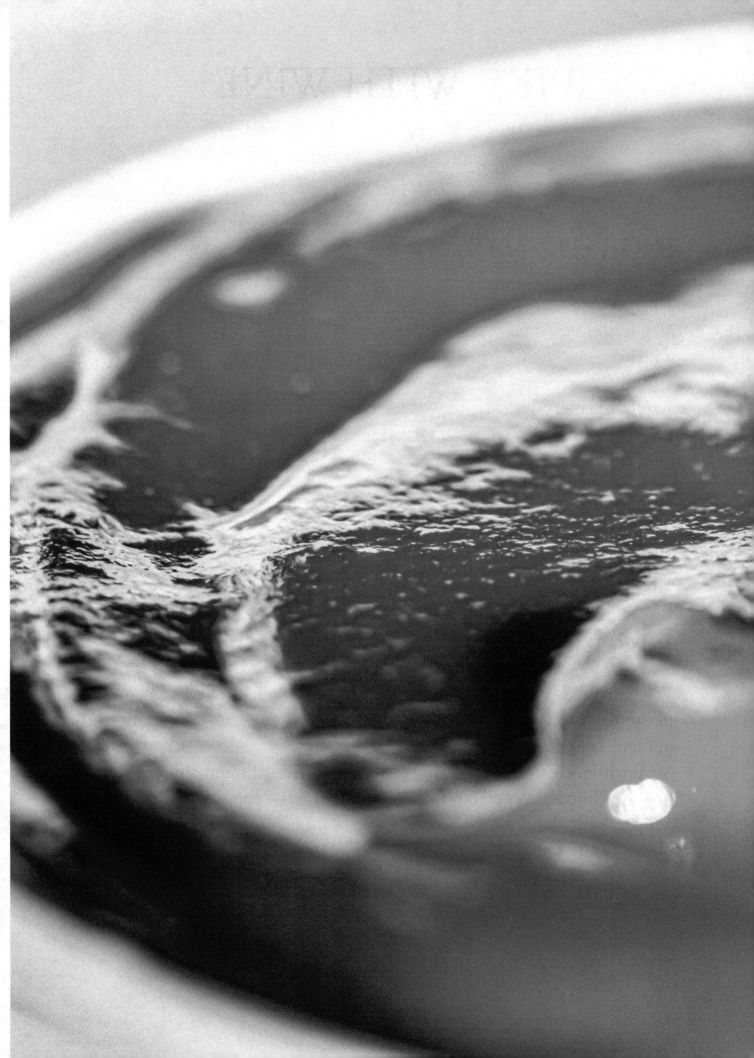

TOMATO SAUCE

INGREDIENTS

1 kg of tomatoes
3 cloves of garlic
oil
salt and pepper
1 onion
1 sprig of basil
5-6 slices of wholemeal bread
1/2 stock cube
1 liter of water

INSTRUCTIONS

Peel the tomatoes after soaking them for a couple of minutes in boiling water. Squeeze the tomatoes to remove seeds, cut them into small pieces, and put them in a pot to simmer for 10 minutes. In a saucepan, put the oil and garlic and finely sliced onion. Add the basil. Cut the bread into squares and add in the pan with salt and pepper. Add the tomatoes and boil for another 20 minutes. Remove the sprig of basil and garlic and add half a liter of hot water. Boil for 8 minutes more. The sauce must be slightly dense.

16

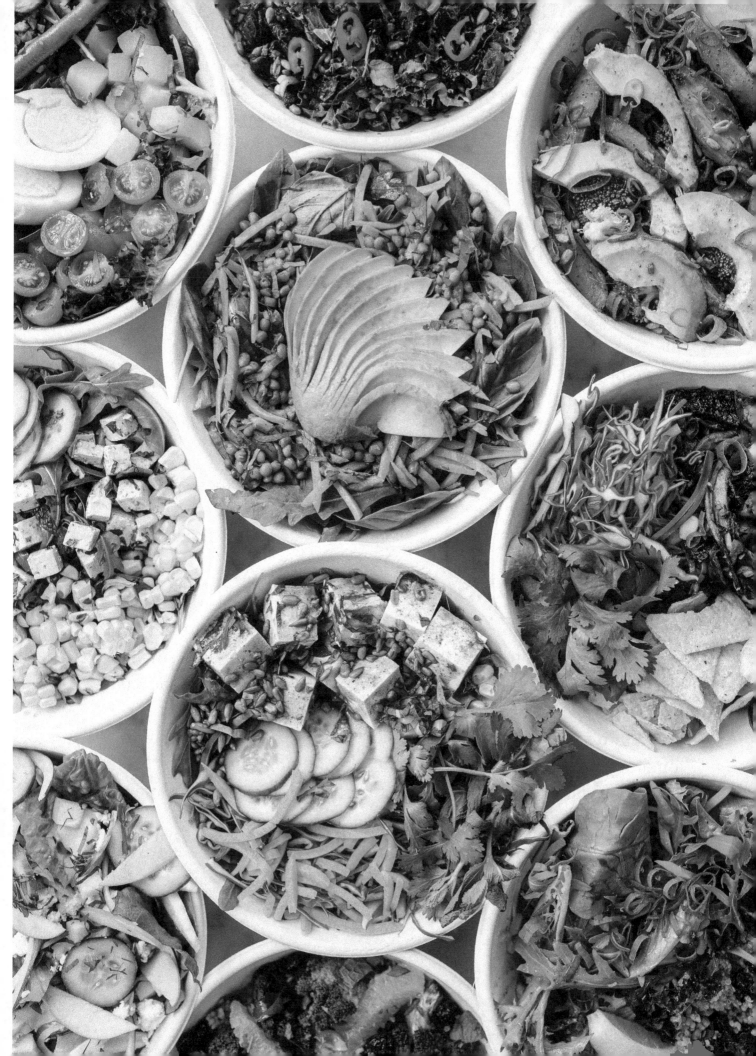

COD WITH VEGETABLES

INGREDIENTS

500 g of cod fillet
2 domes
200 gr of carrots
200 gr of zucchini
1 bell pepper
1 pinch of thyme
1 bay leaf
5 tablespoons of oil
salt and pepper

INSTRUCTIONS

Cut the vegetables into pieces, slice the onions and fry everything in a saucepan with the thyme, bay leaves, salt, 1 tablespoon of oil, and 1 cup of water for 15 minutes. Cut the cod fillet into four parts, arrange it on the cooked vegetables, add more oil, cover the pot, and let it boil for another 20 minutes. Serve with brown rice.

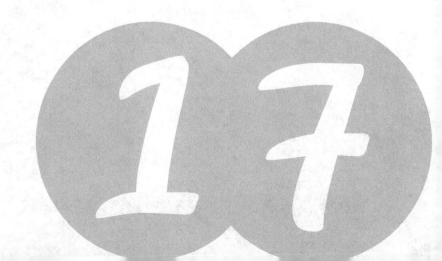

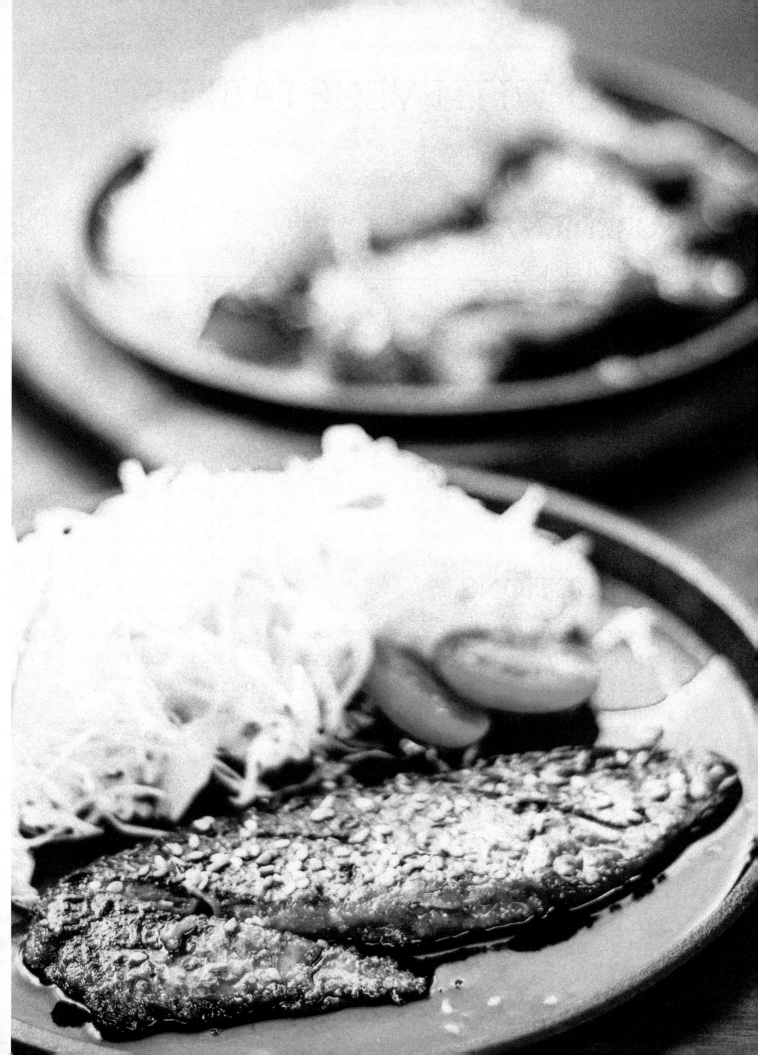

EEL WITH MUSHROOMS

INGREDIENTS

SERVINGS 4

READY IN 30 MIN

800 g of eel
1 onion
2 tablespoons of
chopped parsley
300 g mushrooms
1 cup of white wine
2 tablespoons of olive oil
2 cups of broth
salt and pepper

INSTRUCTIONS

Clean, peel and cut the fish into small pieces (approx. 5 cm). Put the finely chopped onion in the pan with oil and parsley for a couple of minutes. Add fish and brown it until golden. Add the white wine and let it evaporate, then add salt, pepper, and well cleaned and sliced mushrooms. Add the broth and cover. Cook until the fish is done and serve hot.

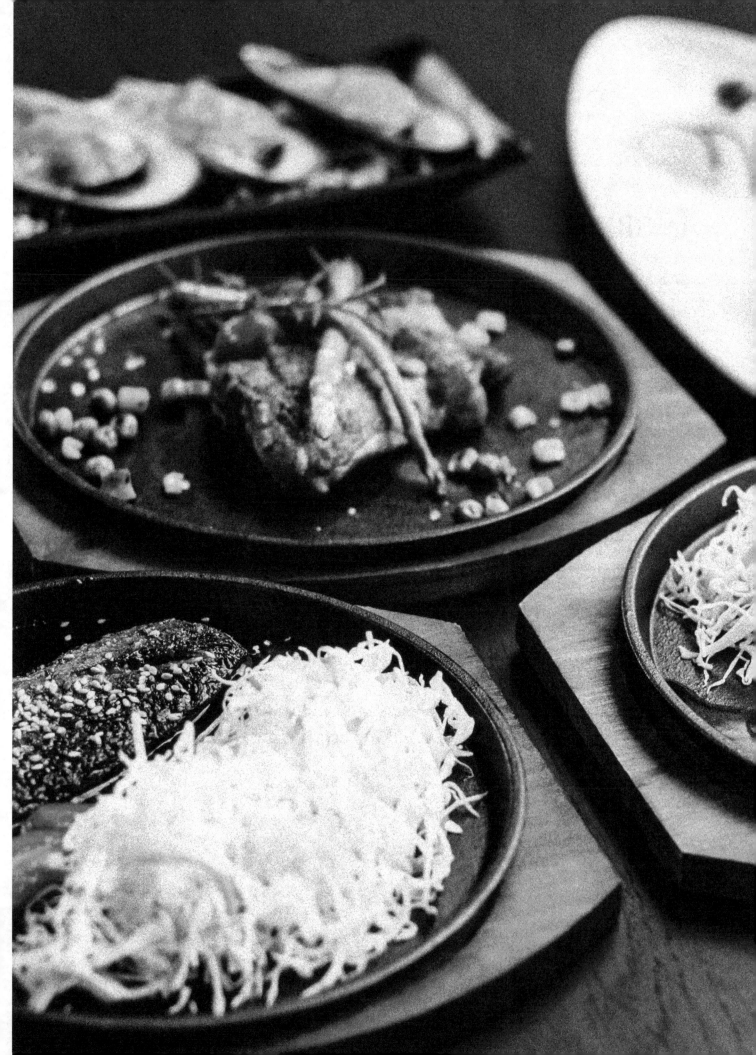

FISH STEW

INGREDIENTS

SERVINGS 4

READY IN 1 HOUR

1 large eel
1 fish S. Peter
1 redfish
3 squid
1 cup of peeled and
chopped tomatoes
1/2 onion
2 slices of lemon
Laurel
curry
salt and pepper
1 sprig of rosemary

INSTRUCTIONS

Clean the fish, remove the bones, clean and cut the eel into 4 cm, and wash and empty the squid. Make a broth with the fish bones, boiling it with bay leaves, lemon slices, salt, and pepper. Also, add the squid and boil everything in the pot for about 20 min.

Flour the fish, and eel finely chop the onion and fry in the oil until soft and brown. Add a teaspoon of curry and chopped rosemary salt and add the tomatoes. Boil for a few minutes, then adds the squid cut into rounds and the filtered fish soup. Boil over low heat for about 20 minutes. Serve hot with polenta.

19

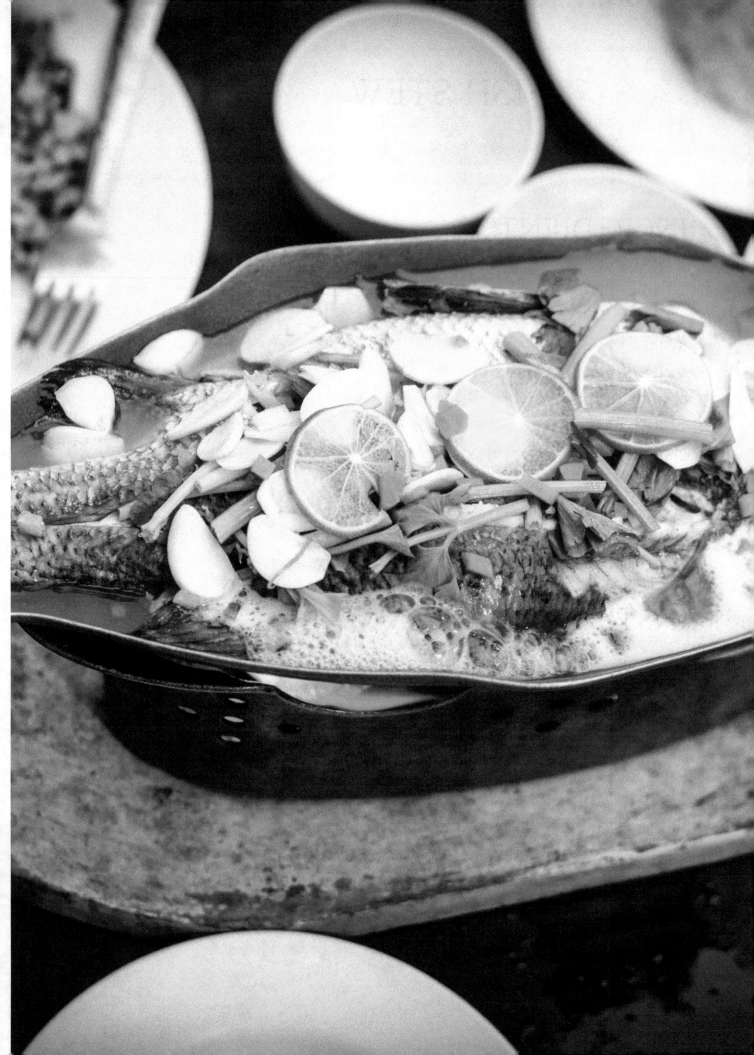

STUFFED SEA BASS

INGREDIENTS

1 kg sea bass
50 g butter
1 cup of white
wine
breadcrumbs
soaked in milk
1 boiled egg
onion
parsley
thyme bay leaf
garlic
salt
pepper
50 gr gruyere
cheese

SERVINGS 4

READY IN 40 MIN

INSTRUCTIONS

Clean and wash the sea bass, then salt it and add pepper. Cut along the back and open that it will be possible to put the filling in. Soak the breadcrumbs in milk, squeeze it, and put it in the bowl. Add the boiled egg, parsley, garlic, and chopped onion. Lightly salt the mixture and fill the sea bass with it. Thinly slice the Gruyere cheese and arrange the slices on the top of the filling. Cover the fish and sew it together. Put the fish, butter, thyme, and bay leaves in a saucepan and sprinkle with wine. Close the pot and leave it on low heat for about 25 min. Serve with the sauce and boiled potatoes.

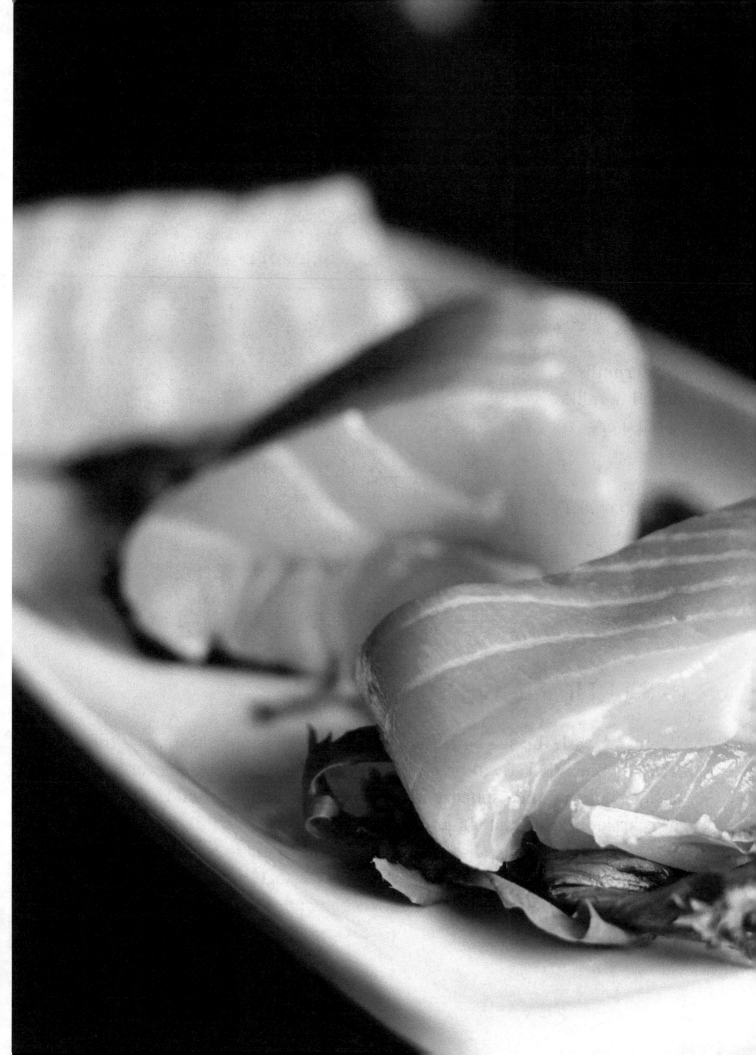

CAKE OF ANCHOVIES

INGREDIENTS

800 gr of anchovies
2 slices of bread
milk water
2 spoons of grated Parmesan cheese
1 tablespoon of grated pecorino cheese
2 fresh but ripe tomatoes
oil
chopped garlic and parsley
broth

SERVINGS 4

READY IN 1 HOUR

INSTRUCTIONS

Clean the anchovies and take the bones out. Soak the bread in milk and water. Squeeze them and put them in a bowl; add parmesan and pecorino cheese, garlic, chopped parsley, and mix everything. Grease the pan with oil and put a layer of mixture and a layer of lightly salted anchovies, and continue with another layer until all the ingredients are used up. Finish with anchovies covered with salted and peppered; tomato slices, then add a pinch of oregano. Add two cups of broth and close the pot. Over low heat, simmer for 30 minutes. Serve still hot.

21

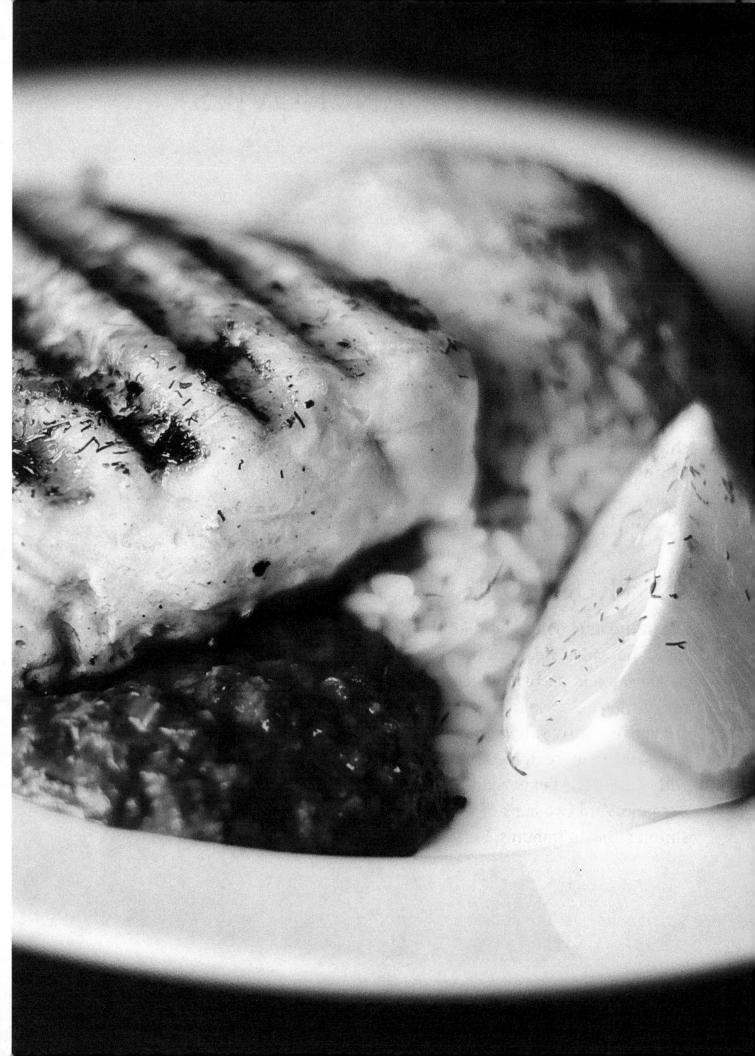

CUTTLEFISH IN WET

INGREDIENTS

SERVINGS 4

READY IN 1 HOUR

1 kg of cuttlefish
1 clove of garlic
1/2 tablespoon of chopped parsley
1 cup of broth
1/2 cup of peeled and chopped tomatoes
salt and pepper
2 tablespoons breadcrumbs
oil

INSTRUCTIONS

Clean the cuttlefish and cut them into rather large pieces, then put them in the pot with the oil, the chopped parsley and garlic, salt and pepper, and two tablespoons of breadcrumbs, cover and leave until the water contained in the cuttlefish has evaporated. Add the chopped tomatoes and the broth, then cover and let it boil for about 30 minutes. Add broth if necessary while cooking.

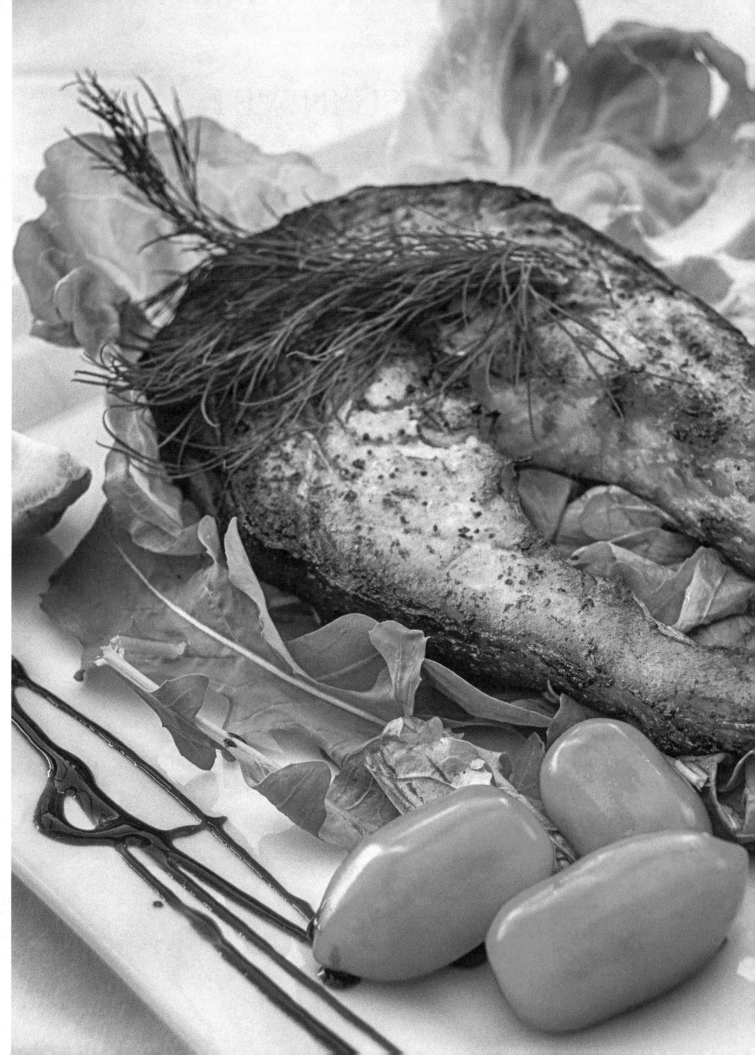

FISH ROLLS

INGREDIENTS

SERVINGS 4

READY IN 40 MIN

4 fillets of sole or other fish

1 sprig of parsley

10 mussels

salt and pepper

30 gr butter

2 tablespoon ful of breadcrumbs

1 tablespoonful of cream

1 lemon

1 tablespoon of white wine vinegar

1 egg white

INSTRUCTIONS

Wash and dry the fillets and cut them in half if they are too big. Open the mussels and finely chop them. Mix them in a bowl with the cream, egg white, breadcrumbs, salt, and pepper. Mix well and spread some of this mixture on the fish fillets. Roll them up and tie them with kitchen string. Put them in a pot, sprinkle them with lemon juice and salt and pepper. Fry them over low heat for 20 minutes. Chop the parsley very fine and fry it in a pan with butter and salt. Remove the rolls, remove the string, place them on a hot serving dish and sprinkle with fried butter and parsley.

23

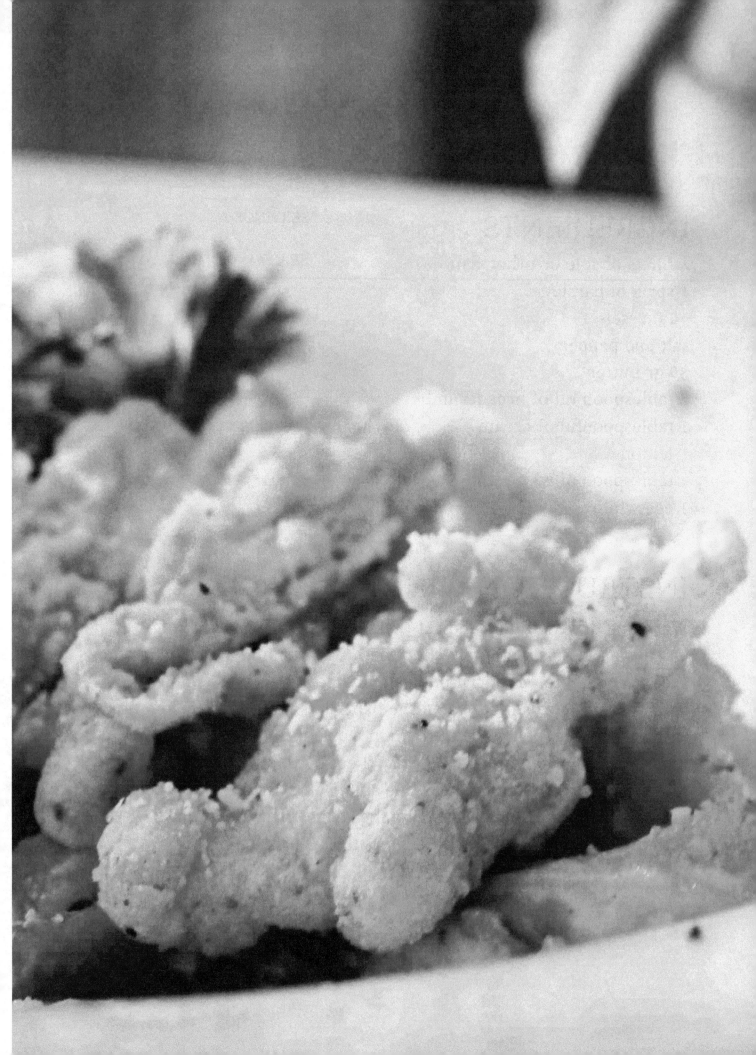

MULLETS ROLLS

INGREDIENTS

SERVINGS 4

READY IN 1 HOUR

4 mullets
chopped garlic
parsley
polymer clay
Oregano
5 green olives
1 tablespoon of capers
salt and pepper
breadcrumbs
oil
laurel

INSTRUCTIONS

Clean the mullets, wash and dry them. Put the garlic, parsley, thyme, and oregano in a bowl add a few tablespoons of oil, pitted and chopped green olives together with the capers. Mix well.

Take 4 pieces of foil, grease them, sprinkle with breadcrumbs. On each mullet put a little mixture of olives and bay leaves and salt. Wrap the mullets in the tinfoil, close them and place them on a baking sheet. Bake in the oven at 180 C for about 30 minutes.

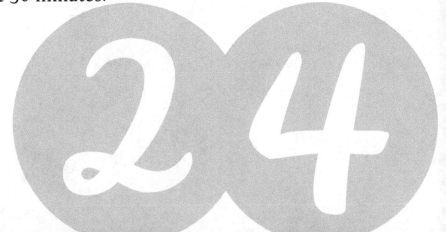

24

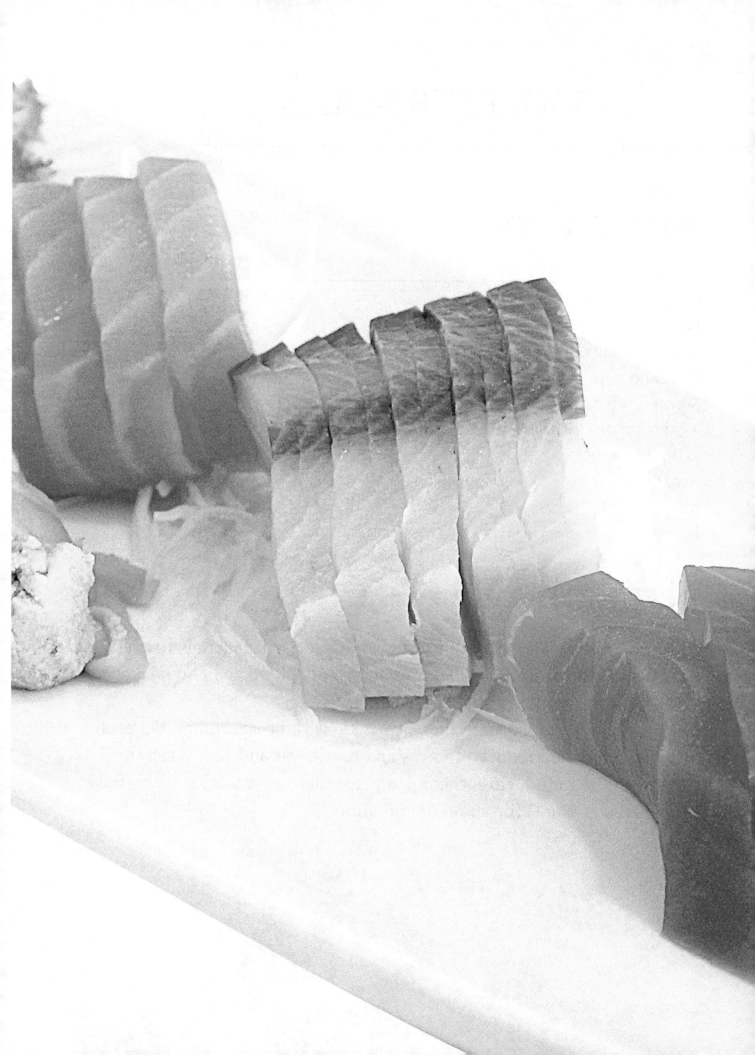

CPSIA information can be obtained
at www.ICGtesting.com
Printed in the USA
BVHW012335291121
622518BV00031B/242